Guidelines for Home Rehabilitation of Your Dog:

After Surgery for Torn Knee Ligament

First Four Weeks, Basic Edition

Deborah Carroll
CSCS, CCRP

GRACE IS EVERYWHERE

REHABILITATION AND CONDITIONING FOR ANIMALS

PREFACE

Some of the information contained in this volume has been published previously by me on my various websites beginning in January, 2007. Until this particular current publication, the one you are reading, I have had available on my various sites (and on some sites that co-opted the material) a general outline for the first four weeks of post-surgical or post-injury rehab because the demand for this information has been so great. As of now, the updated content of this volume is not available on any of my websites.

When I first began publishing a simple home-based plan to the internet it was only a four-week, progressive walking exercise plan, useful for a variety of rehab situations. Online and where I live and work, I found that most pet caretakers were told to keep an animal crated until a certain point, somewhere between four and twelve weeks after injury or surgery. They were then usually told to either "return to normal activity" or "gradually increase walks".

Since I came from a studious background of writing training programs for professional athletes, friends, and neighbors, I knew that an outline with a more definite recipe was needed to guide caretakers toward better healing and functional rehabilitation for companion animals. People really need to know more about what to do at home with their pet after surgery.

An introductory, four-week version of return to activity is what is contained in this booklet. What has happened though over time is that I have encountered many situations wherein people have interpreted my basic instructions in contrary ways. This means they often omit bits they

1

thought they could "get away with omitting", and often they have done that in a way that has been detrimental to the pet.

Therefore, what this booklet also contains is a little more descriptive explanation of how to enact a basic and successful home-based rehab plan well for weeks one through four …and to enact it simply. There is no "bullet point" version of this booklet, because bullet points will not describe the details of functional rehab enough so that the animal receives more benefit while receiving less harm or discomfort. This has been my experience in my practice with humans and other animals.

Many people have received a "bullet point" version as discharge instructions from the vet, yet they find they really would like more instruction after they get home and the drama begins to calm.

Most people are overwhelmed after their pet is injured. After they have visited the vet to find out about the injury and potentially the pet has even received surgery; caretakers often do not recall much of what was said in the clinic as instruction. Some discharge instructions also contain recommendations that caretakers are to perform actions with the pet that the people don't actually know how to perform safely or well.

This booklet is a basic edition, hoping to remedy some of the early confusion. It is also the closest you may come to bullet points from me outside of my professional website. There will also be an expanded edition, which contains more in-depth looks at potential pitfalls and additional remedies, along with greater explanation as to why I believe some therapies are better than others, especially for wellness and healing complementary to a home environment.

Thank you, on behalf of your pet, for taking this time to learn more about the healing methods available for them.

Table of Contents

PROLOGUE

This info is actually written for people just like any of you! I go into homes of people who are baffled about how to enact rehab care for their pets, and I try to bridge the gap, explaining what needs be done in comparison and contrast to a lot of ideas they've collected from many sources.

I suggest that if you read this book you don't skip around, and don't skip the Preface or any other part of the book...it's not a romance novel or sci-fi adventure, so every part is "the good part", of course.

You **do** need to be able to understand and follow instructions contained in this volume. They are very simple instructions, yet each one has purpose; purpose in the times and amounts and types of work I have chosen.

There is a little room for negligence or inability, however cutting corners on purpose while reading the directions or while performing the work will not bring about the best results possible. Accidental negligence or learning curve mistakes often work out okay, because people see and understand their mistake and make corrections. Usually cutting corners on purpose brings fairly mediocre results and may even result in further injury to your pet. I have definitely collected a lot of data via interaction with clients, as well as via my own life choices and subsequent outcomes to be able to present a great case against corner-cutting!

HOW TO USE THIS HOMEWORK GUIDE

Read the Preface.

Read the Prologue.

Read the whole booklet before beginning the work.

Thank you! Now continue to read this chapter. The above three bullet point sentences were for people who really want bullet points. Both the Preface and the Prologue contain beneficial information, and I think the following contents will answer several questions you might not even know you have!

This homework covers guidelines that may be used after any invasive procedure performed for surgical repair of your pet's knee after a torn ligament, whether any of the bones were cut or not. Right now it does not matter so much that you know exactly which surgery was performed; the restrictions and care are equally beneficial.

These guidelines are also very beneficial for recovery after surgery for torn meniscus and after surgical intervention for osteochondritis dissecans (OCD) (yes, really, but different from psych OCD) of the stifle (knee) joint. Whichever method of surgery was used, this homework is an excellent place to continue the healing journey!

As I stated earlier, written programs like this were not readily available, if at all, when I first began working officially in small animal veterinary medicine rehab in 2004. I knew from working with athletes and others, as well as from reading related research for several decades, that very slowly progressing, return-to-function programs were needed for our pets, as well.

In light of what I knew, I began using simple post-surgical protocol I developed. The larger discussion, continually, is among varieties of veterinarians who have come to believe in a particular method or methods of surgery to be used to stabilize the knee after ruptured cranial cruciate ligament. Regardless of method used, this intro protocol should be very beneficial toward accustoming the joint to greater amounts of use again, toward improving bone healing, and toward improving bone and muscle strength.

I don't have the money to fund a large study or the time to ask for it at this point or in recent years. I do, however, have the validation of many veterinarians who have seen the progress of the pets whose caretakers have fastidiously followed my instruction for at least 8 weeks.

Often people see such notable improvement after only 4 weeks that they don't understand the need to continue to follow through with progressive rehab. In well-established human rehabilitation protocol for ACL surgery, patients are progressed through criteria-based functional activities and evaluations for discharge from rehab are targeted between 4 and 6 months after surgery[1].

Is this happening with your pet?

My preference is that people follow at least 12 weeks of rehab protocol for their pets in almost every case. The feedback from situations of which I am aware where this has occurred has been entirely positive. This homework is an excellent place to continue the healing journey, so take a deep breath and move forward confidently!

Also, as noted, my practice and protocol are based on using the home or a standard vet clinic environment to accomplish functional rehabilitation. I prefer land-based exercise because I find it very practical for most pets and their caretakers after this surgery. You may put your internet researching skills to good use by looking for research data which encourages the use of weight-bearing exercise, where possible, to bring about greatest changes toward healing, including bone strengthening and the strengthening of soft tissue, as well as muscle hypertrophy. The latter is often the reason animals are referred to me; people want to see the muscle rebuilt where it has diminished over time due to injury and subsequent lameness (muscle atrophy).

Some people will want to utilize a clinic and a water treadmill in addition to the instructions in this booklet, possibly because the clinic option is available and their veterinarian has recommended it. Most people do not have the option of a rehabilitation facility for their pet, and that's okay, because it's not necessary to have that in order for your pet to recover...so don't fret!

Regardless, I find that people are really in need of instructions that outline steps they may take to assist the healing and improved return to function of their pet in the home environment. Caretakers usually just don't know what to do that is proactive and practical at home after pet surgery.

I also emphasize over and over that pain control is important to my (or any) rehab protocol. If you are not going to use enough pain control to help your pet bear weight on the injured leg, then you should consider using the water treadmill.. The only potential advantage the treadmill has over land-based exercise and drills is that it lessens the weight of the animal, therefore reducing the need for pain medication.

Regardless, your pet spends most of its time outside of the treadmill, if you choose to utilize one, and the need for adequate pain medication stands. Subsequently most people find that with enough pain control, the pet uses the injured limb, so let's use these instructions to help them return to using it well.

It is extremely important for pet caretakers to learn how to control and care for their companions at home after this surgery whether or not they also entrust this aftercare to a clinic for a few hours a week as well.

Do collaborate with your vet clinic, yet also learn how to do your part, hopefully aided by the ideas in this booklet.

[1]You may find out more about the topic of clinic-based human rehabilitation from books like Postsurgical Rehabilitation Guidelines for the Orthopedic Clinician, Hospital for Special Surgery, Department of Rehabilitation, Copyright 2006, Elsevier, Inc.

SOME RESTRICTIONS

First and foremost: pay attention to the discharge instructions your veterinarian and I are giving you regarding *confinement during the times your pet is not doing the controlled, constructive work outlined in this homework*. Please pay special attention to the part about *no running, jumping, or playing*.

Our goal is to minimize impact on the knee so that the inflammation will subside and additional damage will not occur. This "additional damage" could easily include the destruction of the surgery!

If your veterinarian did not say so, please note there should *not* be any flying over couches or galloping stairs, no jumping *into* or *out of* cars and trucks, no jumping *onto* couches or your bed, likewise no jumping *off of* couches or beds, no twisting very fast in tight circles or sliding on ice, or freedom in and out of doggie doors. No owner jumping out from behind things to scare the dog into running crazy funny around the house like you sometimes like to do.

"No running" really means no running...not to the door when the doorbell rings, no running away from Halloween costumes, no running from one end of the house to the kitchen every time the fridge or a plastic bag is opened, no running to your location when you yell to ask the dog if it wants to go outside, and no running inside after the ball, which is *very* similar to no running *outside* after the ball.

No, **no swimming** until at least 8 weeks after this surgery and then only if no lameness is present. Swimming does not usually add quality to the rehabilitation of hind limbs after knee surgery, while the time expended and potential for additional injury are great. Your time is better spent on other activities, with the exception of about 2% of cases that have extenuating circumstances. Not everyone can be in the 2%, so for now, assume that your pet is not in the 2%. I intend to discuss this further in the expanded edition. This booklet is the basic edition.

I do **not advise** or promote the use of **passive range of motion** (PROM) after this surgery. There are **many** reasons for this, and a few of them are as follows: you run a greater chance of injuring your pet and/or the surgery if you do PROM. It should become clear that when appropriate pain control measures are implemented and there are no additional damages or complications, your pet will bend and flex, sit, stretch, etc…in increasing amounts.

If they are allowed to increase flexion and extension on their own, without our forcing the issue and causing them greater pain, my experience is that they will do so when they are given appropriate pain control medications. I have seen hundreds of cases resolve with good function and gait and without PROM being put upon them by me or anyone else. Again, if they are not bending the leg or standing on the leg well, the reason is most likely pain, so please pay special attention to the pain chapters in this booklet.

Please know that *completely* restricting your pet after this surgery, as in confined to a cage and only out to potty a couple of times per day, is not proved to be the best method for encouraging overall healing for an injured body. The focus to this statement is that complete restriction can be much more harmful than good, depending on the injury and the caretaker.

On the other hand, if you are not going to follow restrictions, both in the home and on walks, then your pet may be better off left in the crate!

Our goal is to allow for healing by not allowing dynamic, concussive activity (bouncing, running, jumping), and by encouraging appropriate, easy, progressive exercise that you control. This slow, progressive exercise will allow the joint to become accustomed again to bearing loads. It will also encourage use of the operated leg, which will, in turn, encourage the development of the type of stabilizing scar tissue we want around the knee.

This approach to rehab will also use the best tools available, a progressive program, medication, and gravity, to build muscle as the operated leg use is increased.

If your veterinarian has recommended cage rest only, then please see if they will read this short booklet and agree to the simple concepts. In many cases, you will have been given this booklet by your veterinarian, so no problem. Even with the recommendation of strict cage rest only, a caretaker needs to know how to conduct potty walks, and this plan simply builds from that instruction.

Please also know that if your vet told you to completely restrict and crate your pet for days or even weeks after this surgery, that was likely because vets, including specialists, (and also rehab practitioners) are accustomed to seeing people allow their pets to completely destroy a surgery that might have otherwise been dealt with easily and conservatively. The destruction of the surgery occurs when someone allows the pet to do the things I told you not to do (and more) in the earlier paragraphs in this section. Please use your best judgment and these guidelines, and ask questions if you are unsure about whether or not to do an activity. A simple recovery time is a short 12 weeks, so try to keep on track and it will be accomplished before you know it!

I am the middle person here, and I'm hoping with this booklet for you to build a base of good, solid activity that promotes healing, as I have been doing in person in my practice for years. I have a background in sports therapy, physical recovery, surgical recovery, etc., for humans as well as for animals, and I have been working in collaboration with veterinarians for many years.

This plan will only work for everyone's benefit if you follow both the **guarded exercise AND the thoughtful restrictions**, follow both the parts you *want to* as well as those bits that are for your pets own good, even if you *don't want to* (E-collar! Reduce food! Use a Harness! Restrict!).

I come into the mix in order to guide you and give you instructions about how to safely encourage healing using structured exercises and proven methods. "Structured exercises" means you have to be *in control* and *use control* to help your animal follow the plan and heal. "Proven methods" covers ideas like reducing the amount of food you are feeding, regardless of your psychological resistance to it, so that you don't add extra fat to the burden of healing!

I **highly recommend** using a harness to do all of the exercises and drills I present in this book. Please do this so that you may better accomplish controlled exercises without putting the extra stress on your pet's neck that a collar alone would put on it.

Rehabilitation works when a slowly progressive and structured plan is followed. Loose guidelines rarely ever work well for the long run and never work as well as a thoughtful, structured plan.

WEEK 1

WHEN TO BEGIN

Week 1 of active homework may usually be safely begun three to five days after surgery *if* you are taking thoughtful, attentive care of your pet and of the surgical site, as well as paying attention to the recommendations in this booklet regarding restrictions, medications, and rechecks with your veterinarian.

I believe general rehabilitation begins the moment the pet caretaker/owner/client, walks out of the clinic with their pet after diagnosis or surgery. This is one reason I have made productive instructions available on the Web for years and am now working to make this more informative home guide available.

It is my observation that most people do not hear the discharge instructions given to them at the time they collect their pet from the clinic after a stay regarding injury or surgery or illness of any complicated variety. People are understandably concerned for their pet and frightened about not knowing how to best care for them. The exchange seems to go something like this:

*Discharge Tech: "...and you need to make sure you keep on the e-collar, day and night, except when Snugglepumpkin is eating, until you return for suture removal."

*Client hears from tech: "...glah blattity blah...",

*Client hears in their own head and may even say out loud, "OMG!!! POOR SNUGGLEPUMPKIN!! WHAT ARE WE GOING TO DO!!? POOR BABY!! ARE YOU OK??? DOES THAT HURT?????"

*Discharge Tech: "Did you understand all of that?" (after about a 15 minute discourse on the do's and don'ts).

*Client: "What? Um, yes. Are we done?"

This dialogue story not meant to slight the client or caretaker in any way! It has merely been my experience that people are fearful of not knowing how their pet feels and how to best help them. This fear seems to take over their brains and eat up most serenity, especially if the caretaker is unfamiliar with medical conditions and procedures.

Another scenario is also played out all too often, and that is one wherein the client is listening attentively yet for whatever reason not a lot of instruction is given out from the clinic at discharge, when the caretaker collects the pet. Hopefully this booklet will help in either of these or any similar situations.

AT HOME...NOW WHAT?

Many people are really at a loss as to how to care for their pet once they get them home (or back to wherever they are going outside of the clinic), even if they did hear well-delivered discharge instructions and believe they understood every word.

I find in my practice that there are a lot of questions and complications that arise once everyday living is encountered outside the vet's office, and that's when the snags can really trip healing. Most people have no idea what issues they will encounter with the pet after surgery.

Many veterinarians will suggest that rehab work may begin at suture/staple removal, when your vet sees the pet again roughly 10-14 days after surgery and examines the surgical repair site.

If a vet is recommending that you wait to do exercise until after suture removal , that is often based on their wanting to see the healing that has occurred and perhaps see if discharge instructions they gave to you are being followed. There is quite a bit of non-compliance among caretakers regarding the use of e-collars and restrictions in the home, and therefore there is a relative complication or failure rate with surgeries. No one wants that for your pet!

A lot of vets also think of rehab in terms of how they are accustomed to it being presented at conferences, usually involving a water treadmill, some balls, balance boards, and a clinical setting. That is only one possible form of potential rehab.

Many times the "standard" recommendation to begin rehab at suture removal is because the wound should be well-sealed by that time, and it is recommended to wait until the incision site is sealed before putting the pet into the water for treadmill work.

My rehab protocol begins well before suture removal, as I previously mentioned, because you need to know how to best care for your pet in an active home environment. I encourage you to do your best to show your veterinarian, and your pet, that you are capable of this level of care.

Vets may also think starting rehab involves some degree of concussive, joint-jarring exercise that the pet is not ready to perform. This booklet introduces successful, relatively peaceful, alternatives to those high-impact scenarios.

NO WATER TREADMILL??

The water treadmill is a tool that may be used, however I don't find it necessary in order to encourage or achieve recovery from this surgery for small animals. Large animals, like horses, seem to benefit greatly from water work, especially since pain control is difficult and medication balance is often complicated for horses.

In cases of heavy animals with injuries or surgeries, the water treadmill is potentially a great benefit toward healing, since it can relieve weight and pressure when adequate pharmaceutical pain control cannot be achieved. With the use of water in these cases, the animal will use the leg and bear weight on it, thus progressing muscle growth (hypertrophy) and joint use.

And, as always, a well-written, progressive program of action that follows principles of exercise physiology and training needs to be pursued to achieve the most benefit, whether on dry land or in the water.

Since I have had experience working with animals in water treadmills as well as with athletes in the field, it has been easy for me to design and implement successful home-based rehabilitation programs that teach pet caretakers how to encourage physical healing and functional rehabilitation beyond injury and surgery. It is also therefore easy for me to give productive guidelines that assist in home care. Additionally, I have dealt with my own multiple injuries and surgeries, as well as those of other humans, and I'm always comparing and contrasting feedback and outcomes with a variety of animals!

WALKING WORK

Week 1 exercises consist of 2-4 five minute walks only per day. I purposely buried this instruction among lots of previous information so you wouldn't speed ahead and only get half the info!

Also, if you are finding these exercises today and your pet had surgery four weeks ago (or four months ago) yet hasn't ever begun at the basics and isn't using their affected leg well, please begin at Week 1 to follow this homework successfully and establish a good base.

Another bullet point: There should be at least two-hours of rest in-between each walk session.

All walks in my guidelines should be done *very slowly* so as to encourage more equal weight bearing on all limbs and especially on the surgery limb. When the animal goes too fast, they can "cheat" and not use the surgery leg much or well. Speedy walks could also prolong the inflammation and pain as well as damage the knee even more.

The knee joint needs to be protected from concussive activity right now, activity that puts an abrupt pressure on the joint. I have described the slow walk pace as wedding march (without the step pauses), funeral dirge, or as a client recently said, "wagon walk", which I found super funny (picture Pioneers trudging across Kansas and Oklahoma or any barren outback).

Again, the recommended harness will greatly assist with accomplishing slow, controlled walks. You should also keep your pet walking right next to you, on a short leash. I prefer clipping the leash to the part of the harness that goes across the back of the pet, and that way it is easy to keep them close to me as well as stabilize them if they stumble.

Note: outside sniffing for four minutes and walking for one minute does not constitute the weight-bearing, purposeful exercise we hope to accomplish. Please keep your pet moving consistently, yet slowly, during the controlled exercise drill portion.

These walks are to be *purposeful* exercise and are *separate from potty walks*. Potty walks during this recovery time should be done by going out, getting business done as soon as possible, then coming back in, separate from the five-minute walks. Potty walks should **also** *only be done on the leash*, for control and to keep any surprise clown acts from happening..

I often am able to encourage caretakers in their home or their pet's usual environment to use certain nearby helps to keep the walks moving. For instance, in a neighborhood with streets that aren't very busy with traffic or other dogs, this may mean walking in the street, against traffic flow and away from grass smells. In some areas it is illegal to walk in the street if a useable sidewalk exists. If you live in such an area, then you should learn to use the harness for control, keeping your pet close to your body to perform these slow walks and so that they don't get to stop and sniff every few steps (or at all) if you have to walk on the sidewalks.

PRECAUTIONS AND NOTICING PROBLEMS

Your pet needs to build a base of continual exercise via consistent, non-stop use of the affected limb in the manner I am outlining. This is important for healing, for strengthening the joint and the connective tissue, and for overall success.

Please do not make the mistake of increasing their activity too quickly. You will be able to relate better to this advice if you have had extensive surgery on your own person! If you have had surgery, remember what that felt like, if you can! The body has to have time to adapt, the capillaries need to heal, and just because your faithful dog *will* run a mile with you two weeks after surgery or *will* charge out the door after the cat across the street does NOT mean they *should*, nor are they healed from this surgery…far from it.

Please **stop exercises** for the day if you go to do the next set and your dog will no longer use the leg. Please stop if the leg tissue is more swollen, if the joint is more swollen, or your pet is more lame in another manner.

18

Some animals become lame, for instance, on the front end while compensating for injury to the back end. This would indicate a separate injury your veterinarian should address.

Become accustomed to feeling the size of both knees to determine if there is a difference in size between the surgery one and the other, whether only one knee had surgery or they both did. I suggest that you kneel behind your pet while they are standing, with them facing forward, and you cup your palms around both knees at the same time. Only cup lightly, and move your hands up and down the knee area. You should be able to feel the joint slightly swollen after surgery, and that would be normal.

If there is *more* swelling several days after returning home and/or *more* lameness after walks or additional lameness the next morning, use the time you would normally be using to walk to instead apply ice to the bulk of the knee. For now, some instructions for this are located on my website. If your dog continues to be lame **and** they've had their medication, *allow them to rest and just do potty walks for the day.*

Do call your veterinarian if there is greater pain than when they discharged your pet after surgery, especially if you are giving your pet pain medications and antibiotics. There is more info on pain in a future chapter.

Do call your veterinarian if you happen to know of an incident like the ones listed in the first few paragraphs of "How to Use This Homework Guide" that could have caused an injury to the repair site and especially if your pet is more lame after any incident(s), known or suspected! I'm pretty sure some pets do jumping jacks in their crates…

DOES THIS WORK CAUSE PAIN?

I have not had a pet become more lame strictly as a result of doing the exercises as I have written them or outlined them to clients. This is because these four weeks are very, very basic and slowly progressive. Any continued or additional lameness has been due to other circumstances, and the walks have occasionally uncovered these preexisting problems.

What I'm saying is that the work outlined thus far is so simple and gentle that in itself, it is not going to be damaging under the circumstances we are discussing. In the beginning, this work is hardly more than what is needed to see your pet to the bathroom, which is another skill you will need at home! Greater lameness at this point is therefore usually because of a pre-existing condition that may need further veterinary attention. I cover more about this in the pain chapter.

If your pet continues to hold up their leg more than 3 days after surgery, please read my chapter on pain again and see your veterinarian for appropriate medications. Additional helps include laser therapy, chiropractic, nutrition, and acupuncture to help fight more against the pain and therefore against the limping. In most cases, pain is the cause of limping. I also highly recommend to my clients a form of massage that is represented in a video on my website.

Other beneficial remedies for pain exist as well (Reiki, T-touch, aromatherapy, magnets, etc...), and I find different ones of these to be beneficial at different times to different bodies. Not all body systems respond in the same way to all medications and therapies.

Moreover, I work to get caretakers involved in the most practical therapies for their situation. Often clients want to spend time and money on therapies that I would put further down the list because the most simple, inexpensive, and practical measures have not been yet accomplished.

Out of hundreds of cases, many of them with several complications, I have seen great success in taking a calm approach and starting at the beginning of my protocol. Along the way we may add a variety of helps, and if we stick with the basics up front, we will better be able to understand the nature of deeper problems, if they truly exist.

It has also been my experience that pharmaceutical medications, where available, are hands-down the best post-surgical and post-injury method of pain relief. This is possibly primarily because most other therapies take expertise and/or time and/or money that most of my clients just don't have.

I work to help people realize practicality and try to weigh importance of each activity against available resources (time, money) to get some good things going for their pet's rehabilitation.

I want patients to be as pain-free as possible to begin and continue the homework. *The time for weaning off the drugs is after exercises are accomplished well and healing is progressing solidly and continually*, when the pet is at most graded a one out of four on the lameness scale.

When your pet is doing okay without medications, this is also a great time to rely more on adjunctive therapies, additional helps to take the place of medications if possible. If the pet isn't relieved of pain enough to be able to perform well on this basic four week plan, then your pet will not be ready to advance to the next four weeks of drills and harder work, weeks five through eight.

In some very few situations I have encountered a pet that will not or cannot, for a number of reasons and extenuating circumstances, use their operated limb(s) well after surgery. I discuss some potential reasons for this in the pain chapter.

With a slowly progressing plan, controlled and structured activity may begin sooner than suture removal. You may progress so long as adequate pain control has been achieved. I also hope that your veterinarian understands and is in agreement with this work. They will surely recognize the principles if they have ever trained their bodies or recovered from a surgery!

Your vet may be aware of similar work I've been publishing to the web regarding these guidelines since 2007. *Please share this info with your vet if they are not aware of it and bring them into the mix for continued success.* I have seen many variations of the programs I've written being given out in clinics and used as guidelines for use after injury or surgery, so your vet may be aware of and may already be using similar, descriptive protocol.

DOES LIMPING=PAIN?

SHOULD MY DOG STILL BE LIMPING?

This is the most common question I receive on my website, and the most common answers I give are as follows, based on what I have found to be true in my practice:

If your pet is limping it is most very likely your pet is in pain.

This is easy to say from my current perspective because most of the animals I see are not receiving much, if any, pain medication and/or they are doing too much activity too soon after injury and surgery.

When your pet is limping after surgery, they are not limping solely "because he/she had surgery" per se; the pet is usually limping because he/she is painful after surgery or after an injury. Sometimes I find that people don't associate the two events, meaning they often think that injury equals limping, but they don't know to think that limping usually equals pain.

Overall body pain even occurs with "regular" injuries, since we all compensate for our painful parts by overusing the good parts, making lots of painful parts. Think about situations where this has happened to you, if you can; an injury and the length of time it took for related pain to resolve. Think about any associated pain you had in other parts of your body from compensating for the original pain. Yes, your pet feels similar pain, too.

I DON'T THINK HE'S IN ANY PAIN...

My pain guidelines are true for the majority of the animals I see that are lame and for which someone has said, "I don't think he/she's in any pain". I have had hundreds of cases on which to test this assessment and the theory that pain is not always well recognized.

Working on these cases along with veterinarians to increase pharmaceutical pain control has often proved to us what may seem to be at first only theoretical ideas. Animals formerly reluctant to use their leg *almost always* (roughly 98% of them) begin using the injured limb, usually fairly easily, when they achieve appropriate pain control and activity control. This means more medications and less activity. Reminder: once you have reduced the pain by using medications or other methods, *do not allow* free reign if you intend to continue healing!

ISN'T IT GOING TO HURT HER TO USE THE LEG?

Using an injured leg is not a bad thing; using an injured leg inappropriately, too harshly, with too much force, *is* a bad thing. We want the pet to use the injured leg, yet in the right way. I also want them to use it with help for the pain that using it may cause.

We are not bluntly forcing use here; we are allowing the pet to use the leg when they are comfortable with the level of pain control and functional help that is being offered. There is no need to force use when pain is relieved in almost every case I've encountered after this surgery.

Your pet will also be painful for a while even if they don't have surgery, and surgery is *not* an easier recovery with regard to pain or some other issues. Surgery is not a "restriction-free", "rehab-free", quicker fix.

Some dogs are definitely poor candidates for surgery solely based on their excitable disposition and the difficulty the caretakers have in controlling them, both in the home and on the leash. If you have a pet like this, you may also be able to use over-the-counter or prescription medications to keep them more calm during the recovery time. Ask your veterinarian about these options if necessary.

We want them to use the leg(s) in a correct manner that we dictate, and not use it to do jumping jacks in the crate when you're not looking.

BUT HE FEELS BETTER!!

A fairly widespread misconception is that if they act like they feel better, the pet *is* better, all healed. The reality is that this is not exactly true. This thinking usually subsequently leads people to allow more activity than should be allowed sooner than should be allowed and usually results in messing up your pet again! Just say no to more activity and be content that they do finally feel a little better!

One reason I designed the program the way I did is to keep your pet and you entertained at first, so that no one "gets bored" and beneficial activity and healing may be accomplished. Take advantage of the program design to stay appropriately active while helping the body to heal.

PSYCHOLOGICAL ISSUE?

Limping and leg disuse are also rarely, if at all, psychological issues in my experience. I find that leg disuse does not often (1%?) have to do with the pet psychologically holding back, however it is commonly thought and taught that this is the case. Giving your pet enough pain medication almost always disproves the "psych disuse" theory.

The idea is often presented that the pet has not used the limb for so long that a psychological factor has taken over and they are "just not accustomed to using it" or "just don't want to use it". For most orthopedic surgery cases, I simply find that slowing down the walk speed and giving enough pain medication brings them to use the injured leg.

I have only occasionally and rarely found this idea (psychological disuse) to be true in my practice when dealing with this surgery. I disagree with the premise that most of the patients have become accustomed to not using it, and therefore aren't using it.

The patients I see that are most often not using their legs and that often eventually learn to use them are the ones that have had back surgery, but that is another booklet topic!

Even in the more difficult cases, when a completely out-of-the-usual pharmaceutical pain management protocol was needed, along with a very basic version of my exercise protocol, these animals, too, used their limbs better, more consistently, and often eventually completely.

24

My finding is that if they "just don't want to use the leg" it is because they are in pain when they do use it, except in some few cases like I cover ahead.

I'VE TRIED ALL THAT!

A few possible issues can inhibit limb use after injury, especially if some time has passed since the injury and if little or no definitive functional rehab program has been followed. These issues could include limb restriction due to a buildup of the wrong type of scar tissue or due to contracture. In a couple of cases, formerly undiscovered buckshot or pellets have caused more pain that interfered with recovery.

Persistent pain while on at least two pain medications might equal another x-ray, and that's how we often find the funky stuff that defies our original efforts of rehab and pain control.

I've also had cases where the injury that was diagnosed defied all practical methods of rehab at our disposal and that turned out to have 1) a rare nerve sheath tumor, 2) a pelvic tumor, and 3) a variety of similar, rare issues. More and different x-rays eventually showed some of these things to us. It took a CT scan or MRI to show the tumors. These conditions are more rare, though.

I have had a couple of cases with some very difficult issues to overcome, and I can say that they have, at the least, seemed to become more comfortable with increased and specific rehab and medication intervention, even when their lameness-due-to-very-complicated-circumstances continued over the years.

Therefore, I find that with appropriate pain control methods, which include slow and structured return to function activities, like my recommended walk protocol, the pets will begin using their injured leg(s) again, barring a rare and as-yet-undetected event occurring at the same time.

If you haven't tried giving two medications for pain at the same time to a younger dog and sometimes up to three medications for an older dog, then don't jump right to "it's a tumor" in your thoughts!

JUDGING PAIN

A good portion of my daily rehab work is spent trying to determine the level of pain in my clients based on multiple factors. These factors include the patient's response to prescribed daily activity and exercise programs relative to how these drills are actually being performed by the caretakers.

The amount of work accomplished daily may differ, sometimes greatly, from the type and amount I prescribed. It's important to communicate well while doing this work, especially since a lot of things may go left unsaid when people don't know how important these details might be. If your vet embraces this program of action, then please discuss differences between what is written and what you have actually been doing, especially if there is a setback.

I do this estimation of their feeling pain also contrasting activity against the drugs and supplements the patient is ingesting. I then try to determine whether more veterinary intervention is needed and also the next best course of functional rehab. I review what the vet wrote on the medication label to ensure that we are all on the same page.

Sometimes I find that the pet is not being dosed as much medication as is prescribed on the label. We want to use the medications as a tool in order to get the best results from the rehab work. After substantial improvement, most or all medications can usually be stopped.

If a case seems persistently complicated at this point, I often call or text the vet, sometimes even during my appointment with the pet. The sooner we all work together to get things moving in a beneficial direction, the easier it will be on the pet and subsequently on the people. If you don't have resolution, keep after the solution. I just made that up, and it works.

If the pet is supposed to be doing four walks and is only doing one, and the caretaker thinks the pet is doing great and wants to take them off the meds, this would be ill-advised (barring extenuating circumstances, like other illness or bad reaction to meds). It takes some experience and then some digging to find out that the pet is only doing one walk instead of four sometimes, and my four-walk daily protocol only happens very early on in recovery, so generally speaking it's far too early to reduce meds.

A DAY OF REST

Sometimes the best course of action is *a day of rest*.

Yes, it's possible to over train your pet, just like human athletes over train, and I often see it in my practice, both with humans and with other animals.

I *have* to help pet caretakers understand and deal with the issues of pain and overuse so that the best outcome from injury and rehab may be achieved. This means that the best exercise and drills need to be done in the best manner possible under the circumstances, which means we need to give help to the patient toward getting rid of pain, whether with medications, rest, massage, or any of a variety of helps.

Sometimes *two days of rest* are a substantial remedy, especially if the joints are swollen inside (effused). Effusion often occurs due to too much activity after injury or surgery. Sometimes it's a sign of infection.

When increased effusion occurs, after 1-3 days of rest, I usually start the pet and person back at the beginning of the protocol if the swelling has lessened. If the swelling hasn't lessened with strict rest after a day or two, then have your veterinarian take a look.

You're not losing ground if you didn't really gain it in the first place, so starting back at the beginning is a good thing in some situations. If you did seem to gain ground before a setback, then accept the down time as part of the process, and pick up again with good resolve.

ABNORMAL BEHAVIOR

Be thoughtful about any of your pet's abnormal behavior at home and be communicative to your pet's vet about this behavior; don't wait for questions to be asked, because vets aren't usually mind readers! Pets usually aren't quite acting themselves in the clinic when they see the vet, so I often find that the vet might not have noticed signs like constant panting (while in air condition on a cool floor), since a lot of pets are nervous at the vet and panting regardless. That panting could be a sign of pain. Speak up for your pet.

Maybe the pet caretaker didn't bring up in conversation with the vet some signs of pain that have been seen around the house, and therefore the vet isn't aware that the pet needs more meds or therapy for pain. Again, limping is most often indicating pain.

Snapping at a sibling pet or anyone else if your pet is bumped is often a sign of pain (unless your pet is always a grouch) (except that I've seen some "always a grouch" pets that have actually "always" been in pain).

When I can see a pet acting out of the norm in their home environment, that tells me a lot, and I can convey my concerns to the caretaker and to the vet. Don't hesitate to voice your concerns, should you have them, and let your regular vet know about limping and/or pain.

HOW LONG WILL SHE NEED MEDICATION?

I find that veterinarians with whom I frequently work are noticing the benefit of dosing pain medications for more than just 1-2 weeks after injury so that the pet will use their leg in my rehab programs, and I'm seeing more productive rehab activity in return. The pets do use their legs better, every time we get the combo of pain relief correct (and if there's nothing additional going on, as I've mentioned).

Combos of pain relief could include medications, supplements, and adjunctive therapies. Leg use during a land-based exercise program substantially strengthens the affected areas as well as the whole body under usual (and some unusual) circumstances, and with newfound strength and muscle support, most pets will continue to improve or do well with reduced the pain control interventions.

TORN MENISCUS PAIN

Another sometimes confusing issue that I occasionally see diagnosed after the torn ligament and that is causing additional pain is a torn meniscus. It's confusing because the most common sign in an un-operated leg is a clicking noise. Actually, the most common sign is probably pain, but when we already know we are dealing with the possible pain of a torn ligament, it may not be obvious right away that there is also a torn meniscus. If there is no audible clicking to obviously indicate a torn meniscus, the reason for that could be due to the knee being effused, or swollen, inside the joint.

Effusion displaces knee parts, simply speaking, and doesn't allow for audible clicking, since the parts won't be rubbing on one another if they are pushed apart or away from one another due to swelling and the presence of a lot of extra knee juice. Joint fluid and inflammatory process can effuse a damaged joint.

It doesn't seem to take a lot of swelling for us to not be able to hear the clicking. Otherwise, a clicking sound in the damaged knee is one of the most common ways to detect a torn meniscus in the home. Let your vet know if you do hear this noise, and even if you don't hear clicking, your vet may yet be able to diagnose a torn meniscus.

In older dogs that I've worked with for non-surgical help after a torn meniscus, it has been beneficial in my area for the vets to combine a couple of pain meds (like Tramadol and Gabapentin) as well as an anti-inflammatory to get them through the additional pain of torn meniscus (on top of the torn ligament) and on to better weight-bearing and therefore better muscle improvement. This medication intervention does help the dog use the leg so that they can work through the torn meniscus if surgery isn't performed. Other drugs than the ones I mentioned may be used more prevalently in other areas or countries.

THIS STYLE OF REHAB

Pharmaceutical drugs are great tools for helping pursue functional rehabilitation, as are productive massage, laser therapy, and other adjunctive therapies. With their help, the rehabilitation choice of land-based, weight-bearing drills and exercises may be performed well.

Weight-bearing exercise is the most productive way to build bone, bone strength, muscles, and supportive tissue strength. I am not currently citing any research papers that deal with this topic/statement, because this booklet is merely a basic edition of homework protocol. Otherwise, this information about weight-bearing exercise is widely known and volumes of research proofs exist. I have a few papers cited on my website, www.rehabdeb.com as well, if you'd like to look.

My additional anecdotal findings in my rehab practice are that the increased thigh muscle gained through productive, progressive exercise will

29

help support the joint and also improve function. Validating research also exists regarding this information.

At the same time, these exercises help promote the buildup of the right kind of scar tissue we want to also help stabilize the knee. In most of my cases, this rehab program has served to stabilize the joint and encourage healing very well, according to veterinarians reporting back to me. The majority of clients receiving this surgery on their pets will need the specific information I present in this booklet to help them help the pet through everyday home life.

If limping and pain are your pet's issues, stop them from doing too much activity and do read my recommendations for homework. Regardless of how much time has passed since the injury, if there is notable limping, I recommend you begin at week 1 of the guidelines.

DRUG REACTIONS

The most common reactions to medications that I see are vomiting and diarrhea, usually as a result of the pet being given meds, especially anti-inflammatory, without a full meal. Some meds don't need food with them, but anti-inflammatories and antibiotics really do need a meal. Give a full meal, not just some snacky stuff.

I also strongly recommend you feed your pet their medications separately from their regular meal. I suggest a canned version of the food they regularly eat instead of some other common options people use. Using a version of the food your pet already eats will hopefully keep down the intestinal stress I often see in pets that have been given new medications along with a food item that may really disrupt their digestive system.

People (including yours truly at one time) usually think they can just throw the meds in the food bowl along with the meal, but most of the meds are bitter, and another difficult issue I often encounter is the pet that won't eat its food any longer because it's wary of the "stuff" you have put in the bowl with the food.

We need the pet to eat for healing and life and in order to take their meds on a full stomach. This wariness of trickster food will continue to occur, most of the time, even long after you stop putting the meds in their food, so be forewarned. Tramadol is bitter. Cephalexin smells like a sty. The list goes on…so don't do it. Sometimes the pet will eat the food with meds tossed in for a long time before deciding one day they aren't going to eat it any more. I strongly recommend you don't take that chance; I've seen lots of tedious complications arise from this situation.

If you are in possession of drugs for your pet and your pet is limping or not using the leg, then please use the drugs if there are no medical reasons not to do so. Most of the time my clients are not really clear on the concepts of using the drugs as tools to assist in healing and leg use. Using the pain relievers most often brings about a positive change in leg use. My finding is that the appropriate drugs make an enormous difference over 90% of the time.

If your pet has had a bad reaction to any of the drugs given for this surgery, discontinue them, and let your vet know about the reaction as soon as possible. Sometimes this means a trip to the emergency clinic, just to be on the safe side. The most common reactions are vomiting and diarrhea. Other reactions may include allergic response, like shaking of head because ears are itching and filling with goo as a reaction. If you have to stop using the pain relievers you have for your pet, please reduce your pet to the most basic routine, and speak with your vet about getting drugs or pain reduction methods that will work for your pet.

Use rest, restriction, massage, and ice to help relieve pain during any time your pet does not have other pain relievers after injury or surgery. Fish oil, fish or other animal protein containing Omega 3's, joint supplements with a combination of MSM, Glucosamine, and Chondroitin or Green Lipped Mussels are all beneficial, as are natural anti-inflammatories, like turmeric/curcumin, ginger, rosemary, etc… But make sure you include your vet in the decision to add nutraceuticals (nutrition supplements) to your pet's repertoire. In my area the acupuncture vets often give herbs, too, for assistance against pain. I have been scientifically involved with concepts of nutritional supplementation for over 30 years, and I hope to cover nutraceuticals more in-depth in a future, expanded edition of this booklet.

WRAPPING UP PAIN!

Veterinary medicine, on the whole, wasn't consistently teaching that animals felt pain, in so many words, until the 1980's. The topic wasn't well understood in relation to companion animals. Another point to remember is that in human medicine we don't have pain management down to an exact science, and it took a long time for doctors to admit that babies felt pain! Pain management for people who are able to speak or convey in language and signs we are accustomed to understanding isn't a lot better in very many cases than it is for our pet companions. In light of this understanding, please add the understanding that discoveries in pain management are ongoing, and each medical practitioner's understanding of medications and pain management varies, as well.

So overall, your pet is likely not using the leg because it is painful, and there are some very good helps available for your pet, both pharmaceutical and non-pharmaceutical, that usually work well in combination with one another. And don't ever forget that protecting your pet and controlling their walks and activity is one of the best ways to help manage and reduce pain and discomfort, especially if you don't have access to medications.

Those are some basic ideas and guides about pain.

WEEK 2

Week 2 is just like week 1, but the walks are for ten minutes instead of five. Ten minute walks should only be begun if 3-4 five minute (3-4x5 minute) walks are able to be accomplished without producing greater lameness in your pet.

In other words, do not progress to ten minute walks if your pet cannot do at least three separate five-minute walks a day for a week without limping a lot, being very lame.

Due to time constraints and often due to weather (extreme heat or cold, storms) people say they can only get in 1-2 walks daily. I definitely understand this, because where I live, we often have very many days over 100 degrees F during the summer months. People are also very busy, so I work on ideas to help them accomplish home rehab without a lot of complications.

I recommend, again, using the harness and getting the five and ten minute walks accomplished indoors on bad weather days or when it's dark outside, in order to work in 3-4 walks (or even 1-2) daily. Most people are able to accomplish the shorter walks by keeping their pet walking through the house. I truly don't think 5-10 minutes of indoor walking should be mentally or physically challenging, however if anyone ends up doing 15-20 minute protocol indoors, I suggest turning on some music just to keep the humans on track and entertained! I used to do the indoor walk with Great Danes, using a route that circled the kitchen and the living room. It's usually easy to figure out a path through a home to keep the pet moving and getting accustomed to using their leg correctly.

This program is designed to build on progress that is measured simply by you. This is not a program that you should advance each week *if* the progress and desired physical function are not achieved. It is better to stay with five minute walks when an animal is quite lame, and I frequently find this necessary until we can get appropriate pain medications or other helps in place.

"We" in this case usually means a combination of the veterinarian, the caretaker, and I. I realize that many people reading this publication will not have consistent access to a veterinarian, and I have helps for pain control that are non-pharmaceutical noted in the previous chapter. Only move on ahead when it is sensible. Don't cause your pet additional pain when it is within your power to help.

WEEKS 3 & 4

Week 3 consists of only two (2!) walks per day for a length of 15 minutes each. Do not add them together to make one 30 minute walk. I get asked all the time if that's ok. It's not, because you are still to be building a good, solid, slowly-progressing base.

All the other rules and restrictions still apply. Do not begin the 15 minute walks unless your dog is able to do at least three 10 min. walks per day for a week without having greater lameness. If they can do four 10 minute walks, even better.

Week 4 is the same as above (same restrictions, same care, and same control) and the walks are to be twenty minutes in length. 2×20. Continue to keep the walks separated by at least two hours of rest and recovery. At this point, it would be better to separate the walks by 4-6 hours, if possible.

No running, jumping, playing or swimming.

All of the scenarios listed in the first few paragraphs of the "Some Restrictions" chapter have happened in real life to otherwise possibly sensible people. Having any of those scenarios occur has complicated the recovery from injury. Please forgive me if these all seem like obvious no-no's to you; that is why I said the cited incidents happened to people who were possibly (and probably) otherwise sensible.

Injuries to the surgery site and your pet could still occur at this point.

People have told me they took the dog on a leash out front to potty but thought it was ok to be off the leash in the back yard (because it has a fence), especially as they thought the dog was doing better. Keep in mind the purpose of the leash is for control, and I have even seen clients even need to use the leash in the house, which is a good idea for some dogs.

Continue to protect the pet, and everyone will be happier.

MY BACKGROUND AND DEVELOPING THIS REHAB PRACTICE

These successful homework guidelines I've written and used are based on my having over 30 years' experience in sport science and exercise program design, as well as based on a vast amount of related research that I've read and/or heard presented. At this current point in my animal rehab career, the preceding guidelines are also based on my having worked hundreds of cases with this exercise protocol in action.

Through the years of my practice, I've been learning how to combine the best principles of body ecology, repair, and function as well as complex physical training and recovery principles for humans into productive work with other companion animals. These companions simply need beneficial and practical methods to enact some of those centuries-old principles, methods that encourage their natural abilities without forcing the unnatural, without causing fear, and without overworking and causing more damage!

I have worked professionally, collaborating with pet caretakers, veterinarians, and companion animals, in companion animal rehabilitation since 2004. I began my formal animal rehabilitation career at a veterinary specialty hospital at the request of one of the surgeons there, after she observed for several years some of my attempts to rehab my Great Dane, Grace, who had a LOT of orthopedic issues and subsequently entertained many surgeries and interventions.

My biggest surprise after coming into veterinary rehabilitation was to discover that no well-described, structured, dynamically-progressive, return-

37

to-function plans existed of the sort I was accustomed to seeing and developing for sport and athletic training.

If programs like that were "out there" somewhere, I didn't find them, either on the internet or in the texts that I read in 2004. I also thought I knew that racing horses had sport training programs, as professional athletes, and I had just assumed there was a trickle-down effect to small animal medicine. Maybe you've thought the same. I promptly set about to write some functional rehabilitation training protocol in bite-sized, structured plans that would be simple and hopefully easy to introduce to my clients.

In addition to building the rehab department for the hospital and developing procedure and protocol to use at the time, I made it a point to attend every orthopedic and neurological problem consult that I could, listening to the specialists and the pet caretakers...and learning even more, through practice, about listening to the pets. I got to participate in a great number of consults on a wide variety of problems, and often I was given the opportunity during the consult to explain how I thought my intervention could contribute toward healing. Evidently this mirrored elements of an intense internship, and thankfully the construct fed my learning strengths.

In 2005, I became a graduate of the Certified Canine Rehabilitation Practitioner (CCRP) program offered through collaboration with the University of Tennessee School of Veterinary Medicine and the North Carolina State University School of Veterinary Medicine.

I slowly began to work out my own "what if we did it this way?" and "how can I make that happen better?" questions and answers. I was able to do this regularly, because in addition to having a broad background in sport training and recovery, I am also a Certified Strength and Conditioning Specialist (CSCS) through the National Strength and Conditioning Association. This is the designation one needs in order to be the strength coach for a professional sports team, as an example, for those of you unfamiliar with the organization.

I believe that my study and work for several decades in human sport science has really been the foundation to produce the informative action protocol that exists in the following pages. I combine that "old" yet ever-increasing knowledge with new findings in neuroscience, sport performance, therapeutic remedies, and information I pick up from being active in the veterinary medical community. I believe the result is a practical and medically-informed approach to companion animal rehab that nearly anyone may accomplish!

Additionally, many of the people I have encountered through the internet via my websites or social media that are in need of animal rehab information do not have access to a standard animal rehabilitation clinic. Many of these same people do not even live in close relation to the veterinarian they have used to diagnose and treat their pet, so a definitive guide for home-based rehab is needed.

I have developed the guidelines in this book for use in my mobile animal rehabilitation practice so that I and/or pet caretakers may practice them in the home or any other environment conducive to the work (clinic, barn, quiet park, mountaintop…) in order to rehab their pets after injury and/or surgery. No special tools or equipment are needed for the majority of the exercises and drills I utilize on a daily basis and present in this book..

I do my rehabilitation work as much as possible in collaboration with veterinarians, and it is my strong suggestion that you do the same where a veterinarian is available. I understand that many people reading this guide will have travelled a great distance to obtain surgery for their pet, and they may not have veterinary care nearby. Sometimes when I work long distance with people in similar situations I've also worked to help them find a specialist for their often complicated cases. No one person has all the answers, and collaboration is a great tool. You just don't know what you don't know.

If you have difficulty understanding the concepts in this guide, and you are not close to a veterinarian, yet you have access to a physiotherapist of some sort, an athletic trainer, or a coach (just to name a few other related vocations), then perhaps one of those persons could assist in your understanding any concepts that are presented here and not easily understood by you.

Thank you!

UNTIL NEXT TIME...

This concludes conservative rehabilitation basic instructions for the first four weeks after surgery. This is the bite-sized version, with an expanded edition to follow. For additional information, please see my website, at www.rehabdeb.com.

Thank you very much, again, for purchasing this volume. Spread the word, so that the common-sense ideas in this volume may be introduced to others. And keep it simple. Your pet will read stress off of you, so don't stress and do set about to walk through this guide step by step.

Blessings-
Deborah

ABOUT THE AUTHOR

I have a website at www.rehabdeb.com, a rehab page on Facebook, a Twitter account under rehabdeb, and a presence on LinkedIn. I randomly post super important info or pictures of animals trying to enjoy rehab.

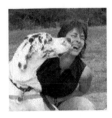

91013868R00027

Made in the USA
Middletown, DE
27 September 2018